# Ketogenic Diet:

# Healthy and Delicious Low-Carb, High-Fat Recipes for Weight Loss

© Copyright 2017 by Kay Grant - All rights reserved.

This document is geared towards providing exact and reliable information in regards to the topic and issue covered. The publication is sold with the idea that the publisher is not required to render accounting, officially permitted, or otherwise, qualified services. If advice is necessary, legal or professional, a practiced individual in the profession should be ordered.

- From a Declaration of Principles which was accepted and approved equally by a Committee of the American Bar Association and a Committee of Publishers and Associations.

In no way is it legal to reproduce, duplicate, or transmit any part of this document in either electronic means or in printed format. Recording of this publication is strictly prohibited and any storage of this document is not allowed unless with written permission from the publisher. All rights reserved.

The information provided herein is stated to be truthful and consistent, in that any liability, in terms of inattention or otherwise, by any usage or abuse of any policies, processes, or directions contained within is the solitary and utter responsibility of the recipient reader. Under no circumstances will any legal responsibility or blame be held against the publisher for any reparation, damages, or monetary loss due to the information herein, either directly or indirectly.

Respective authors own all copyrights not held by the publisher.

The information herein is offered for informational purposes solely, and is universal as so. The presentation of the information is without contract or any type of guarantee assurance.

The trademarks that are used are without any consent, and the publication of the trademark is without permission or backing by the trademark owner. All trademarks and brands within this book are for clarifying purposes only and are the owned by the owners themselves, not affiliated with this document.

# Introduction

I want to thank you and congratulate you for reading my book, *"Ketogenic Diet: Healthy and Delicious Low-Carb, High-Fat Recipes for Weight Loss"*.

This book contains proven steps and strategies on how to lose weight and feel healthier with the ketogenic diet.

The ketogenic diet is, without a doubt, one of the most popular diets of all times. The thought of eating so much fat probably horrifies many of you but the right combination of the right fats, the right proteins and the right carbohydrates has been scientifically proven to work.

The main aim of my book is to provide you with a taster of what you can enjoy on the Ketogenic diet, a selection of delicious recipes that anyone can cook and everyone can enjoy. You will learn the benefits of this diet along with what to watch out for on the negative side and then we'll dive straight into the kitchen.

Thanks again for purchasing this book, I hope you enjoy it!

Contents

Ketogenic Diet:

Healthy and Delicious Low-Carb, High-Fat Recipes for Weight Loss

Introduction

Chapter 1: Ketogenic 101

    The Benefits of the Ketogenic Diet

    The Negative Effects

    Foods to Eat

Chapter 2: Breakfast

    Zucchini and Walnut Bread

    Lemon Raspberry Sweet Rolls

    Ricotta and Blueberry Pancakes

    Breakfast Sausage Casserole

    Cheddar and Sage Waffles

Chapter 3: Lunch

    Caramelized Onion Prosciutto and Parmesan Braid

    Sausage and Kale Soup

    Chicken and Broccoli Zucchini Boats

    Ham and Apple Flatbread

    Mixed Green Spring Salad

Chapter 4: Dinner

Skillet Chicken with Creamy Greens

Slow-Cooker Steak Chili

Sausage and Cabbage Skillet

Creamy Crab and Zucchini Casserole

Slow Cooker Chicken Tikka Masala

Chapter 5: Dessert

Raspberry Pavlova

Lemon Poppy Soufflé

Peanut Butter Chocolate Tarts

Pumpkin Fudge

Mascarpone Cheese Mousse with Berries

Conclusion

# Chapter 1: Ketogenic 101

The ketogenic diet is a low carbohydrate, high-fat diet. To be successful, you must reduce your intake of carbohydrates significantly and replace it with fat. Not just any fat, though; it must be the right fat, the good fats and yes, they do exist. When you cut out the bad carbohydrates and reduce your intake drastically, it will put your body into a state known as ketosis. This is a natural metabolic state whereby your body stops burning glucose for energy (because there isn't any) and starts to burn fat instead. It will also convert fat in your liver into ketones, which are a great source of brain energy.

## The Benefits of the Ketogenic Diet

Ketogenic, or keto, diets have several fantastic benefits and the main ones include:

### 1. Never being hungry again

Ketogenic diets automatically reduce your appetite because you are eating more fat and more protein, both of which lead to increased satiety and fewer calories.

### 2. Lose more weight

Because you are taking in fewer calories and because your body is burning fat as energy, your weight will drop with ease. Also, keto diets tend to remove excess amounts of water from the body resulting in a fast weight loss almost immediately.

### 3. Bye Bye Belly Fat

You have more than one type of fat in your body and it is where the fat is stored that determines your health and disease risks. Visceral fat is the most dangerous and this is stored in the belly – this is fat that must go because it settles around your internal organs. This leads to an increase in inflammation and a resistance to insulin. Most of the fat lost on a keto diet comes from the belly.

### 4. **Down the Triglycerides**

These are fat molecules and higher levels of fasting triglycerides lead to a higher risk of heart disease. Cutting the bad carbs helps to lower that level significantly.

### 5. **Up the HDL**

High-density lipoprotein or HDL is the good cholesterol, the proteins that are responsible for carrying fat to your liver. From there it is either re-used or it is excreted out of your body. The higher your HDL, the lower your risk of heart disease and the only way to do that is to eat plenty of good fat. Add that to a lower triglyceride level and your risk of heart disease plummets.

### 6. **Lower Insulin and Glucose**

Carbohydrates are turned into glucose in your body and these are what raise your blood sugar level. High amounts of blood sugar are poisonous and to counteract that, the body produces insulin. This will cut the blood sugar spike so it doesn't cause any harm. Too much glucose leads to higher levels of insulin and, the more your body produces, the more resistant you become to it. That leads to more insulin and so the cycle goes. This is what can cause type 2 diabetes and by cutting carbs your blood sugar automatically reduces, as does insulin production.

### 7. Blood Pressure Down

Keto diets have been shown to effectively reduce blood pressure, thus lowering the risk of heart disease, kidney failure, and stroke, amongst others.

### 8. Fights Metabolic Syndrome

Metabolic syndrome is a collection of symptoms, including abdominal obesity, high blood pressure, high blood sugar and triglycerides along with low HDL. These symptoms are reduced significantly on the ketogenic diet.

### 9. Better LDL Patterns

Low-density lipoprotein or LDL is the bad cholesterol and too much of the wrong type can cause a higher risk of heart disease. LDL comes in big particles and small ones – a higher level of small particles increases the risk of heart disease while a higher level of big ones decreases it. The ketogenic diet turns small particles into big ones, thus reducing your risks.

## The Negative Effects

Like everything, a ketogenic diet does have some negatives but most of these are short-lived.

### 1. Frequent Urination

This lasts only for the first few days. Because your body is breaking down stored glycogen, water is released into your body and that must go somewhere – the kidneys work hard at removing excess sodium and water from your body, thus you need to pee more!

### 2. Dizzy Spells and Fatigue

With the excess water goes a lot of useful minerals like salt, magnesium, and potassium. Reduced levels can cause light-headedness, headaches, dizzy spells and muscle cramps. Eat more salt or drink salty broth to counteract this, as well as eating plenty of dairy, avocado and leafy green vegetables.

### 3. Hypoglycemia

Or low blood sugar. Your body is used to a certain level of insulin and when your carb intake suddenly drops, so does your blood sugar. Keep an eye on this and see your doctor if it affects you too badly but this should only last for a very short time while your body is adjusting.

### 4. Constipation

The most commonly reported side effect, constipation is caused by dehydration, too little salt, too much dairy or a lack of magnesium. Drink plenty of water, take magnesium supplements and balance your diet accordingly.

### 5. Sugar Cravings

You will experience these because your body has become used to a certain amount of sugar. Don't give in to these cravings because they will pass and don't increase your carbohydrates – too many will feed the sugar craving, strengthening it. Be tough, it won't last for long.

6. **Diarrhea**

Another common side effect that comes from a sudden change in diet or eating too little fat and too much protein. Fat is nothing to fear and you need it so balance your proteins and fats properly.

7. **Ketoacidosis**

This is not a common side effect but it is a dangerous one, more common in those with type 1 diabetes. It is when the body produces too little insulin and can cause you to go into a diabetic coma. Don't push your diet to the extreme by cutting carbs too much and, if you have type 1 diabetes, see your doctor before you start a ketogenic diet.

## Foods to Eat

Most your food intake should be based on these foods:

### Meat and poultry

- Steak
- Red meat
- Bacon
- Sausage
- Turkey
- Chicken
- Duck
- Goose
- Ham

### Fish and seafood

- Salmon
- Trout
- Tuna
- Mackerel
- Prawns
- Shrimp
- Oysters
- Cod
- Halibut
- Sole
- Flounder

**Cheese**

- Cheddar
- Mozzarella
- Gouda
- Edam
- Goat
- Cream
- Blue

**Eggs**

- Any which way you like!

**Cream and butter**

- Grass fed where possible
- Avoid half-fat cream and butter substitutes – eat the real thing

**Nuts and seeds**

- Almonds
- Walnuts

- Pumpkin seed
- Flaxseed
- Chia seed

**Oils and fats**

- Olive oil
- Avocado oil
- Coconut oil
- Avocado
- Guacamole – fresh home made

**Vegetables**

- Leafy green vegetables
- Onions
- Peppers
- Mushrooms
- Tomato
- Cucumber
- Lettuce
- Anything that grows above the ground

**Condiments**

- Salt
- Pepper
- Herbs
- Spices
- Homemade or oil based salad dressings
- Lemon
- Lime

This is not a complete list of foods that you can eat but it encompasses the types of foods. Avoid anything with sugar, refined carbohydrates, pastries, cakes, cookies, vegetables that grow under the ground (apart from onion), anything that says low, no or reduced fat. Stick to whole foods and those that are high in good natural fats and you will see results almost immediately.

The rest of the book is dedicated to some of the most delicious recipes you never thought were healthy to eat!

# Chapter 2: Breakfast

## *Zucchini and Walnut Bread*
**Serves 16**

**Nutritional Information Per Serving**

- Fats – 19g
- Net Carbohydrates – 2.5g
- Protein – 5.6g

**Ingredients:**

- 3 eggs
- ½ cup olive oil
- 1 tsp vanilla extract
- 2 ½ cups almond flour
- ½ tsp salt
- 1 ½ cups erythritol
- 1 ½ tsp baking powder
- ½ tsp nutmeg
- 1 tsp ground cinnamon
- ¼ tsp ground ginger
- 1 cup zucchini, grated
- ½ cup walnuts, chopped

**Instructions:**

1. Preheat your oven to 350° F
2. Whisk the oil, eggs, and vanilla together and set aside
3. Mix the flour, salt, erythritol, baking powder, ginger, cinnamon, and nutmeg together

4. Squeeze excess water from the zucchini through paper towels or cheesecloth
5. Mix the zucchini with the egg mixture
6. Add the dry ingredients gradually, whisking in until blended through
7. Grease a loaf tin, 9x5-inch and spoon the mixture in
8. Cover the top with the walnuts and press in with a spatula
9. Bake for about 60-70 minutes or until cooked through and the walnut crust is browned

## *Lemon Raspberry Sweet Rolls*
**Serves 8**

**Nutritional Information Per Serving:**

- Fats – 25g
- Net carbohydrates – 4g
- Protein – 13g

**Ingredients:**

**Lemon Cream Cheese Filling:**

- 4 oz. cream cheese
- 2 tbsp. butter
- 2 tbsp. erythritol and stevia
- ½ tsp vanilla extract
- 1 tsp lemon extract
- Zest from a large lemon
- 1 tsp lemon juice

**Raspberry Sauce:**

- 2 tbsp. stevia and erythritol
- ¼ tsp xanthan gum
- 1 tbsp. water
- 2 tsp lemon juice
- ½ cup raspberries, frozen

**The Dough:**

- 1 cup finely sieved almond four
- ¼ cup stevia and erythritol
- ¼ tsp xanthan gum
- 1 ¼ tsp baking powder

- 1 egg
- 1 tsp vanilla extract
- 2 cups mozzarella cheese

**Instructions:**

1. Make the cream cheese filling by beating all the ingredients together until smooth
2. Make the sauce by whisking the gum and sweetener together and gradually adding the water and lemon juice. Heat over a medium-low heat and add the raspberries; stir constantly until it begins simmering; remove from the heat and set to one side
3. Preheat your oven to 350° F and great a 9-inch round pan.
4. In a double boiler, bring about 2 inches of water to a simmer and turn the heat down
5. Combine the flour, sweetener, gum and baking powder together and add the extract and egg – whisk to a very thick mixture
6. Add the cheese and place over the boiler; stir continually until the cheese has melted and combined with the flour. It should star to look like proper bread dough
7. Transfer the mixture to a sheet of parchment paper, knead to make sure all the ingredients are combined and then form into a rectangle. Cover with another piece of parchment and roll to a 12x15-inch rectangle
8. Remove the paper and spread the cream cheese over the top, leaving ½-inch all around the edge uncovered

9. Spread the raspberry sauce over the top and then, beginning with a long side, roll it into a log
10. Seal the edges together by pressing and cut the log into 8 slices
11. Arrange the slices in the greased pan and bake until golden-brown, about 24-26 minutes
12. Serve warm or leave to chill

## *Ricotta and Blueberry Pancakes*

**Serves 5**

**Nutritional Information Per Serving:**

- Fats – 22.6g
- Net Carbohydrates – 5.9g
- Protein – 13.4g

**Ingredients:**

- 3 eggs
- ¾ cup ricotta
- ¼ cup vanilla almond milk, unsweetened
- ½ tsp vanilla extract
- 1 cup almond flour
- ½ cup golden flaxseed meal
- 1 tsp baking powder
- ¼ tsp salt
- ¼ cup blueberries
- ¼ - ½ tsp stevia powder

**Instructions:**

1. Preheat a skillet
2. Mix the eggs, vanilla, milk and ricotta together in a blender
3. In another bowl mix the flour, meal, baking powder, salt, and stevia
4. Add the dry ingredients to the blender slowly, blending until you have a smooth batter
5. blend in 2 or 3 blueberries per pancake
6. Melt some butter in the skillet
7. Pour 2 tbsp. batter in and cook, flipping when light brown on one side

8. Repeat with the rest of the batter and serve warm with extra berries

## *Breakfast Sausage Casserole*
**Serves 6**

**Nutritional Information Per Serving:**

- Fats – 42g
- Net carbohydrates – 4.8g
- Protein – 19.2g

**Ingredients:**

- 1 lb. pork sausage
- 2 cups shredded green cabbage
- 2 cups zucchini, peeled and diced
- 3 eggs
- ½ cup mayonnaise
- 2 tsp Dijon mustard
- 1 ½ cups shredded cheddar cheese
- 1 tsp dried sage
- Cayenne pepper for seasoning

**Instructions:**

1. Preheat your oven to 375° F
2. Grease a medium casserole dish
3. Heat a skillet and brown the sausage until almost cooked
4. Add the onion zucchini and cabbage, stirring and cooking until they are tender and the sausage is cooked through
5. Spoon the mixture into the prepared casserole dish
6. Whisk together the eggs, mustard, mayonnaise, pepper and sage to a smooth mixture
7. Add 1 cup of the cheese and stir in

8. Pour the mixture over the casserole and top off with the rest of the cheese
9. Bake for about 30 minutes, or until the cheese has melted and browned lightly
10. Serve immediately

## *Cheddar and Sage Waffles*

**Serves 12**

**Nutritional Information Per Serving:**

- Fats – 17g
- Net carbohydrates – 3.8g
- Protein – 6.5g

**Ingredients:**

- 1 1/3 cup sifted coconut flour
- 3 tsp baking powder
- 1 tsp dried sage
- ½ tsp salt
- ¼ tsp garlic powder
- ½ cup water
- 2 cups coconut milk
- 2 eggs
- 3 tbsp. melted coconut oil
- 1 cup cheddar cheese, shredded

**Instructions:**

1. Heat your waffle iron
2. Whisk the flour, baking powder, and all the seasonings together
3. Add in the liquid ingredients and whisk to a stiff batter
4. Add the cheese, stirring it through
5. Grease the waffle iron pans thoroughly and put 1/3 cup batter onto each section
6. Close and cook until you see steam and the top will open without the waffle sticking

7. Repeat with the rest of the batter and serve hot

# Chapter 3: Lunch

## *Caramelized Onion Prosciutto and Parmesan Braid*
**Serves 6**

**Nutritional Information Per Serving:**

- Fats – 23g
- Net carbohydrates – 5g
- Protein – 21g

**Ingredients:**

- 1 tbsp. butter
- 1 fine chopped medium onion
- 1 crushed garlic clove
- 1 tbsp. balsamic vinegar
- 3 oz. thinly sliced prosciutto
- 2 tbsp. minced fresh basil
- 2 cups fine grated mozzarella
- ¾ cup almond flour
- ½ tsp salt
- 1 egg
- ½ cup + 1 tbsp. grated fine grated parmesan
- Fresh black pepper for seasoning

**Instructions:**

1. Preheat your oven to 375° F
2. Heat a skillet over a medium heat and melt the butter

3. Wait for the foam to stop and then cook the onion. Stir occasionally until the edges have browned and the onions are caramelized
4. Add the garlic and cook for a minute
5. Add the vinegar and cook until it has almost evaporated
6. Add the prosciutto, separating the slices
7. Cook for about a minute, stirring and then add the basil and remove the pan from the heat
8. Season to taste with salt and pepper
9. Prepare a double boiler and bring the water to a simmer
10. Put the cheese, flour, and salt into the top part and stir together
11. Place over the bottom part and heat, stirring, until the cheese has melted and you have a dough ball
12. Put the dough onto a piece of parchment paper and knead it to incorporate everything thoroughly. Pat into an oval shape and cover with another sheet of paper
13. Roll to a rectangle about 14x9-inches, straightening the paper as necessary to stop wrinkles appearing in the dough
14. Spread the onion filling over the middle third of the cheese dough and sprinkle 1/3 cup of parmesan over the top
15. Down the long sides, cut strips of about 1-inch wide and crisscross them over the filling. Fold the ends over before you put the last strips over.

16. Wisk the egg and brush it over the braid. Sprinkle the rest of the parmesan over the top and season with black pepper
17. Bake for about 18-22 minutes or until golden brown
18. Remove from the oven and leave to cool for about 5 minutes before removing the bottom parchment paper and slicing

## *Sausage and Kale Soup*
**Serves 6**

**Nutritional Information Per Serving:**

- Fats – 24g
- Net carbohydrates – 6g
- Protein – 16g

**Ingredients:**

- 1 lb. sweet Italian sausage, ground
- 1 tbsp. butter
- 1 chopped yellow onion
- 1 peeled and diced carrot
- 2 crushed garlic cloves
- 2 tbsp. red wine vinegar
- 1 tsp dried basil
- 1 tsp dried oregano
- 1 tsp dried rubbed sage
- ¼ - ½ tsp crushed red pepper flakes
- 4 cups low-salt chicken broth
- ½ head cauliflower, cut into florets
- 1 cup heavy cream
- 3 cups chopped kale
- ½ - 1 tsp salt
- ½ tsp black pepper

**Instructions:**

1. Heat a large pan over a medium heat and cook the sausage, stirring to break the meat up
2. Cook until cooked through and browned, around 5 minutes and then use a slotted spoon

to remove the sausage. Drain on a paper-towel covered plate and discard the drippings
3. Melt the butter in the same pan and, when it has stopped bubbling, cook the carrot and onion until the onion is translucent and starting to brown on the edges
4. Add the garlic, stir and cook for a minute
5. Add the vinegar and cook until it is syrup, scraping the browned bits off the bottom of the pan
6. Add the herbs and pepper flakes, pour the cream and stock in and turn up the heat
7. When it reaches simmering pint, add the cauliflower and reduce the heat
8. Simmer until the cauliflower is fork-tender, around 10 minutes
9. Add the sausage and kale and cook for another minute or two, until the kale has wilted and the sausage is hot through
10. Season with pepper and salt and serve hot

# *Chicken and Broccoli Zucchini Boats*

**Serves 2**

**Nutritional Information Per Serving:**

- Fats – 34g
- Net carbohydrates – 5g
- Protein – 30g

**Ingredients:**

- 2 large zucchini
- 2 tbsp. butter
- 3 oz. shredded cheddar
- 1 cup broccoli
- 6 oz. cooked chicken, shredded
- 2 tbsp. sour cream
- 1 green onion stalk
- Salt and pepper for seasoning

**Instructions:**

1. Preheat your oven to 400° F
2. Slice the zucchini in half lengthwise and scoop out the flesh. Leave a shell of about ½ - 1 cm thick
3. Melt the butter and pour 1 tbsp. into each boat
4. Season with salt and pepper and cook for about 20 minutes
5. Shred the chicken and cut the broccoli into small bite-sized pieces
6. Combine the chicken and broccoli with the cream, season to taste

7. Take the cooked zucchini boats out of the oven and divide the chicken between them
8. Sprinkle cheese over the top and bake for a further 10 – 15 minutes, until the cheese is melted and started to brown
9. Serve hot garnished with the chopped onion

## *Ham and Apple Flatbread*
**Serves 8**

**Nutritional Information Per Serving:**

- Fats – 20g
- Net carbohydrates – 4g
- Protein – 16g

**Ingredients:**

**The Crust:**

- 2 cups grated mozzarella cheese
- ¾ cup almond flour
- 2 tbsp. cream cheese
- ½ tsp salt
- 1/8 tsp dried thyme

**The Topping:**

- I cup grated Mexican cheese
- ½ small red onion, sliced thinly
- ¼ apple, deseeded and cored – leave the peel on and slice thinly using a vegetable peeler
- 4 oz. ham, cut into chunks
- 1/8 tsp dried thyme
- Salt and pepper for seasoning

**Instructions:**

1. Preheat your oven to 425° F
2. Prepare a double boiler and bring water in the bottom pan to a simmer and then reduce the heat

3. To make the dough, mix the ingredients in the top bowl of the boiler and bring to a simmer; stir to incorporate the ingredients until the cheese has melted and a dough starts to form
4. Take the dough from the bowl and knead it on a piece of parchment paper
5. Roll it into a ball and then flatten into a disc shape. Cover with more paper and roll into a circle of about 12-inches – straighten the paper where necessary
6. Remove the top parchments paper and place the dough, in the second one, in a 12-inch pizza pan
7. Poke holes over it and bake for about 6-8 minutes or until golden brown
8. Remove from the oven and turn the heat down to 350° F
9. Sprinkle ¼ cup of cheese over the cooked dough and arrange the slices of onion
10. Add the apple and then the ham and sprinkle the rest of the cheese over the top
11. Bake for about 5-7 minutes, or until the crust has gone brown and the cheese has melted.
12. Remove from the oven and slide the flatbread off the parchment; cool on a rack for a couple of minutes before slicing

## *Mixed Green Spring Salad*
**Serves 1**

### Nutritional Information Per Serving:

- Fats – 37g
- Net carbohydrates – 4.3g
- Protein – 17g

### Ingredients:

- 2 oz. mixed greens
- 2 tbsp. raspberry vinaigrette
- 3 tbsp. roasted pine nuts
- 2 tbsp. shaved parmesan
- 2 sliced bacon
- Salt and pepper

### Instructions:

1. Cook the bacon until it is crispy
2. Mix all the ingredients together and stir until dressed thoroughly
3. Serve immediately

# Chapter 4: Dinner

## *Skillet Chicken with Creamy Greens*
**Serves 4**

**Nutritional Information Per Serving:**

- Fats – 38g
- Net carbohydrates – 2.6g
- Protein – 18.4g

**Ingredients:**

- 1 lb. boneless chicken thigh, skin on
- 2 tbsp. coconut oil
- 1 cup chicken stock
- 1 cup cream
- 1 tsp Italian herb
- 2 cups leafy greens
- 2 tbsp. butter
- 2 tbsp. coconut flour
- Salt and pepper for seasoning

**Instructions:**

1. Preheat a skillet and melt the coconut oil
2. Season the chicken all over and brown until cooked through with crispy skin
3. While the chicken cooks, make the sauce by melting 2 tbsp. butter in a small pan and whisk in the flour

4. Add the cream and bring to a boil; the sauce should thicken after a couple of minutes so add the herbs
5. Lift the chicken from the pan and set to one side
6. Pour the stock into the pan and stir to deglaze it
7. Whisk the sauce in and add the greens, stirring to coat them
8. Lay the chicken over the top and serve

### *Slow-Cooker Steak Chili*

**Serves 12**

**Nutritional Information Per Serving:**

- Fats – 41.3g
- Net carbohydrates – 5.6g
- Protein – 32.4g

**Ingredients:**

- 2 ½ lb. steak, cut into cubes about 1-inch
- 1 tbsp. chili powder
- ½ tsp cumin powder
- ½ tsp salt
- ¼ tsp cayenne pepper
- 1/8 tsp black pepper
- ½ cup sliced leeks
- 2 cups whole canned tomatoes with juice
- 1 cup beef or chicken broth

**Instructions:**

1. Put all the ingredients into your slow cooker, in the order they are given
2. Stir together, cover and cook on high for about 6 hours or until the steak is tender
3. Shred some of the steaks and break up the tomatoes
4. Serve hot

## *Sausage and Cabbage Skillet*
**Serves 4**

**Nutritional Information Per Serving:**

- Fats – 14.6g
- Net carbohydrates – 3.5g
- Protein – 18.2g

**Ingredients:**

- 4 spicy Italian chicken sausages
- 1 ½ cups shredded green cabbage
- 1 ½ cups shredded purple cabbage
- 12 cup diced onion
- 2 tbsp. coconut oil
- 2 slices Colby Jack cheese
- 2 tbsp. fresh cilantro, chopped

**Instructions:**

1. Remove the sausage casings and chop the meat
2. Melt the coconut oil and cook the onion and cabbage for about 8 minutes, or until tender
3. Add the sausage meat, stir and cook for a further 8 minutes
4. Sprinkle the cheese over the top, cover the skillet and turn off the heat
5. Wait for about 5 minutes, until the cheese has melted then remove the lid and stir
6. Top with cilantro and serve

## *Creamy Crab and Zucchini Casserole*
**Serves 9**

**Nutritional Information Per Serving:**

- Fats – 11.9g
- Net carbohydrates – 2.8g
- Protein – 7.2g

**Ingredients:**

- 3 zucchini
- 1 tbsp. butter
- 1 onion, sliced in half and then thinly sliced
- 1 crushed garlic clove
- 1 tbsp. red wine vinegar
- ½ cup heavy cream
- 4 oz. cream cheese
- 2 tsp Old Bay seasoning
- ½ tsp salt
- ¼ tsp pepper
- 8 oz. crab meat
- 3 thinly sliced green onions
- ½ cup grated Mexican cheese blend

**Instructions:**

1. Preheat the oven to 35° F and grease a 9x9 baking dish
2. Bring water up to a simmer in a steamer
3. Spiralize the zucchini and season with a little salt; steam for about 5-7 minutes
4. Remove the steamer basket and drain off the excess water

5. Heat a large skillet and melt the butter; cook the onions until tender then add the garlic and cook for a further minute
6. Add the vinegar, stir to scrape the pan until the vinegar has almost evaporated
7. Add the cream and the cream cheese and cook until the cheese has melted and the sauce has thickened up; stir constantly
8. Stir the crab and green onion in, and season
9. Add the zucchini spirals, stir to combine and transfer to the baking dish
10. Sprinkle cheese over the top and bake for about 20-25 minutes or until the cheese has melted and is going brown
11. Serve hot

## *Slow Cooker Chicken Tikka Masala*
**Serves 5**

**Nutritional Information Per Serving:**

- Fats – 41.2g
- Net carbohydrates – 5.8g
- Protein – 26g

**Ingredients:**

- 1 ½ lb. chicken thighs, with bone and skin
- 1 lb. boneless, skinless chicken thighs
- 2 tbsp. olive oil
- 2 tsp onion powder
- 3 minced garlic cloves
- 1 inch grated ginger root
- 3 tbsp. tomato paste
- 5 tsp garam masala
- 2 tsp smoked paprika
- 4 tsp salt
- 10 oz. diced canned tomato
- 1 cup heavy cream
- 1 cup coconut milk
- 1 tsp guar gum
- Fresh cilantro for garnishing

**Instructions:**

1. De-bone the chicken and chop all the chicken thighs into small pieces
2. Place in the slow cooker and grate the ginger on top
3. Add the dry spices

4. Add the tomato and paste and mix together well
5. Add ½ cup coconut cream and mix; cover and cook on high for 3 hours or low for 6 hours
6. Add the rest of coconut milk, the cream, guar gum and mix thoroughly
7. Serve hot

# Chapter 5: Dessert

## *Raspberry Pavlova*
**Serves 6**

**Nutritional Information Per Serving:**

- Fats – 15g
- Net carbohydrates – 2.4g
- Protein – 32.g

**Ingredients:**

**The Base:**

- 4 egg whites
- ½ cup erythritol
- 1 tsp vanilla extract
- 1 tsp fresh lemon juice
- 2 tsp xanthan gum

**The Filling:**

- 1 cup heavy cream
- 3 oz. frozen berries

**The Topping:**

- 18 fresh raspberries
- A couple of mint leaves

**Instructions:**

1. Preheat your oven to 300° F
2. Whisk the egg whites until foamy

3. Add in the sweetener gradually, beating until you have stiff peaks
4. Add the lemon juice, vanilla and xanthan gum; fold carefully
5. Place parchment paper on a baking sheet and draw round a bowl or cup 6 times on the paper
6. Spoon the batter onto each circle and use a spoon to create a well in the center of each one
7. Bake for about one hour until the pavlova are golden brown and crispy
8. Leave to cool and make the filling. Blend the berries with the cream until thick – about 3 minutes
9. Spoon the mixture into each pavlova and top off with fresh berries and the mint

## *Lemon Poppy Soufflé*
**Serves 4**

**Nutritional information Per Serving:**

- Fats – 10.8g
- Net carbohydrates – 2.9g
- Proteins – 9g

**Ingredients:**

- 1 cup ricotta
- 2 eggs, separated
- ¼ cup erythritol
- 2 tsp lemon zest
- 1 tbsp. fresh lemon juice
- 1 tsp vanilla extract
- 1 tsp poppy seeds

**Instructions:**

1. Preheat the oven to 350° F
2. Beat the egg whites to a foam and add 2 tbsp. erythritol; beat to a stiff peak
3. Cream the egg yolks, ricotta and the rest of the erythritol in another bowl
4. Add the lemon zest and juice, stir, then add the poppy seeds and vanilla; Stir to combine
5. Fold the whites into the egg yolk carefully
6. Grease 4 small dishes or ramekins and divide the soufflé between them
7. Shale and tap the ramekins gently to flatten the soufflé and bake for about 20 minutes; the top should be set but a little jiggly

8. Serve immediately

## *Peanut Butter Chocolate Tarts*

**Serves 4**

**Nutritional information Per Serving:**

- Fats – 26.8g
- Net carbohydrates – 3.9g
- Protein – 9.8g

**Ingredients:**

**The Crust:**

- ¼ cup ground flaxseed
- 2 tbsp. almond flour
- 1 tbsp. erythritol
- 1 egg white

**The Top Layer:**

- 1 avocado
- 4 tbsp. cocoa powder
- ¼ cup erythritol
- 1/ tsp vanilla extract
- ½ tsp cinnamon
- 2 tbsp. heavy cream

**The Middle Layer:**

- 4 tbsp. peanut butter
- 2 tbsp. butter

**Instructions:**

1. Preheat the oven to 350° F
2. Make the crust by combing all the ingredients together

3. Press it into greased tart pans and smooth it up the sides
4. Bake for about 8 minutes and then leave to cool
5. While it bakes, mix the top layer ingredients together in a blender until smooth
6. Melt the butter and peanut butter and pour it over the crusts
7. Refrigerate for 30 minutes
8. When set, add the top layer, smooth it out and refrigerate for 30 minutes before serving

## *Pumpkin Fudge*
**Serves 25**

**Nutritional Information Per Serving:**

- Fats – 10.6g
- Net carbohydrates – 1.6g
- Protein – 1.2g

**Ingredients:**

- 1 ¾ cup coconut butter
- 1 cup pumpkin puree
- 1 tsp ground cinnamon
- 1 tbsp. coconut oil
- ¼ tsp ground nutmeg

**Instructions:**

1. Line a square baking pan, 8x8 inch, with foil
2. Meth the coconut butter over a low heat
3. Remove from the heat and add the spices and pumpkins; stir well – the mixture should be grainy and thick

4. Add in the coconut oil, stir to make sure everything is combined
5. Spoon the mixture into the pan and spread it evenly
6. Put some wax paper over the top and press the fudge firmly down
7. Take the wax paper off and lift the fudge out of the foil
8. Peel off the foil and slice the fudge into 25
9. Refrigerate until needed

# *Mascarpone Cheese Mousse with Berries*

**Serves 12**

**Nutritional Information Per Serving:**

- Fats – 15.9g
- Net carbohydrates – 3.2g
- Protein – 1.9g

**Ingredients:**

- 8 oz. mascarpone
- 1 cup whipping cream
- 1 pint mixture of berries
- ¾ tsp liquid vanilla stevia

**Instructions:**

1. Whip the cream, mascarpone, and sweetener together until you get stiff peaks
2. Spoon into individual dishes and top off with berries
3. Refrigerate until ready to eat

# Conclusion

Thank you again for reading my book!

I hope this book was able to help you to understand that the ketogenic diet is not bad for you. It isn't like many other diets that are so restrictive that they are boring and impossible to keep up. With the ketogenic diet, you can eat well and you can lose weight as well as feeling healthier and fitter than you have done for a long time.

The next step is to continue your ketogenic journey. Experiment in the kitchen with the foods that you can eat, and banish those that you can't. Learn to enjoy food all over again and push restrictive low-fat diets out of your life forever.

Finally, if you enjoyed this book, then I'd like to ask you for a favor, would you be kind enough to leave a review for this book? It'd be greatly appreciated!

Thank you and good luck!

www.ingramcontent.com/pod-product-compliance
Lightning Source LLC
LaVergne TN
LVHW040202080526
838202LV00042B/3283